30 DAILY PRAYERS FOR DEPRESSED DOCTORS

Uplifting and Inspiring Prayer for Depressed Doctors

Michelle T. Eidson

Introduction

In the fast-paced world of medicine, where tireless dedication meets immense pressure, the weight on a doctor's shoulders can become overwhelming. The constant demands of saving lives, navigating complex cases, and shouldering the responsibility of patients' well-being can take a toll on even the strongest of souls. It is during these challenging moments, when the heaviness seems unbearable, that the power of prayer can provide solace and strength.

"30 Daily Prayers for Depressed Doctors" is designed to accompany you on your path as a medical professional and is filled with prayers that provide solace, courage, and direction. Within the pages of this captivating book, doctors will find respite from the shadows that sometimes cloud their minds. Each prayer is carefully composed, drawing from the depths of empathy, wisdom, and faith to address the unique struggles faced by physicians battling depression. Whether it's the weight of difficult decisions, the emotional toll of witnessing suffering, or the personal challenges that arise from balancing a demanding career with personal well-being, these prayers serve as a beacon of light to guide doctors through their darkest moments.

Don't forget to include your daily prayer request, and then sit back and watch God do what only he can.

DAY 1

Dear God,

As I begin this day, I pray for strength and resilience to face the challenges that come my way. Help me find joy in my work and bring healing to those in need, despite my own struggles.

Prayer Request

_____

_____

_____

_____

DAY 2

Heavenly Father,

I come before you burdened with the weight of depression. Lift my spirits and grant me the clarity of mind to provide the best care for my patients. Renew my passion for medicine and restore my sense of purpose.

Prayer Request

_____

_____

_____

_____

DAY 3

Dear Lord,

In the midst of my own darkness, let me be a beacon of hope for those who feel lost. Give me the wisdom to offer comfort and encouragement to my patients, knowing that healing extends beyond physical ailments.

Prayer Request

DAY 4

Heavenly Father,

Guide my hands as I treat my patients today. Give me the ability to diagnose accurately and the compassion to provide gentle care. Grant me the strength to persevere even when my own spirit feels weak.

Prayer Request

_____

_____

_____

_____

DAY 5

Dear God,

Help me find moments of peace and tranquility amidst the chaos of my profession. Show me the beauty in the miracles of healing that I witness each day, and remind me of the profound impact I have on the lives of others.

Prayer Request

_____

_____

_____

_____

DAY 6

Dear Lord,

I surrender my anxieties and worries to you. Replace them with a sense of calm and assurance that I am capable of overcoming any obstacles I may face. Restore my confidence in my abilities as a doctor.

Prayer Request

_____

_____

_____

_____

DAY 7

Heavenly Father,

Grant me patience and understanding when dealing with difficult patients or challenging situations. Help me respond with kindness and empathy, even when I feel overwhelmed. Fill my heart with compassion.

Prayer Request

DAY 8

Dear God,

I pray for a renewed sense of purpose in my medical career. Remind me of the reasons I chose this path—to make a difference in the lives of others. Give me the strength to persevere and find fulfillment in my work.

Prayer Request

_____

_____

_____

_____

DAY 9

Dear Lord,

When the weight of depression presses upon me, remind me of the healing power of hope. Allow me to see glimmers of light in the lives of my patients, and let their stories inspire me to keep going.

Prayer Request

_____

_____

_____

_____

DAY 10

Heavenly Father,

As I step into the hospital today, shield me from the negativity that surrounds me. Surround me with positivity, encouragement, and support. Help me find joy in the small victories and celebrate each step forward.

Prayer Request

DAY 11

Dear God,

Grant me the courage to seek help and support when I need it. Guide me to resources, whether it be counseling, therapy, or the support of friends and family. Help me find solace in knowing that I am not alone.

Prayer Request

_____

_____

_____

_____

DAY 12

Dear Lord,

When the weight of depression feels unbearable, remind me of the incredible privilege it is to be a doctor. Let gratitude fill my heart as I reflect on the opportunity to impact lives and bring healing to others.

Prayer Request

_____

_____

_____

_____

DAY 13

Heavenly Father,

I pray for resilience in the face of setbacks and failures. Help me learn from my mistakes and grow stronger as a doctor. Give me the determination to persevere, even in the face of adversity.

Prayer Request

DAY 14

Dear God,

Protect my mental and emotional well-being as I navigate the challenges of my profession. Shield me from burnout and guide me towards a healthy work-life balance. Help me prioritize self-care.

Prayer Request

_____

_____

_____

_____

DAY 15

Dear Lord,

Grant me the wisdom to recognize when I need to take a step back and recharge. Give me the courage to set boundaries and prioritize my own mental health. Help me find rest and rejuvenation outside of my medical responsibilities.

Prayer Request

DAY 16

Heavenly Father,

I pray for a network of supportive colleagues who understand the unique challenges we face as doctors. Surround me with compassionate individuals who can offer guidance, empathy, and a listening ear.

Prayer Request

_____

_____

_____

_____

DAY 17

Dear God,

Remind me that it is okay to ask for help and lean on others during difficult times. Let go of my pride and allow me to receive the support and encouragement I need. Strengthen the bonds of friendship and camaraderie among my fellow doctors.

Prayer Request

DAY 18

Dear Lord,

I pray for moments of respite and joy amidst the demands of my profession. Help me find laughter and delight in the simple pleasures of life. Renew my spirit and restore my sense of wonder.

Prayer Request

_____

_____

_____

_____

DAY 19

Heavenly Father,

When I encounter cases that seem hopeless, remind me that miracles can happen. Let me be an instrument of your healing power, and grant me the faith to believe in the impossible.

Prayer Request

_____

_____

_____

_____

DAY 20

Dear God,

Grant me patience and understanding with myself. Help me embrace my imperfections and acknowledge that it is okay to struggle. Fill my heart with self-compassion and remind me that I am doing the best I can.

Prayer Request

_____

_____

_____

_____

DAY 21

Heavenly Father,

I pray for clarity and wisdom in making medical decisions. Help me navigate the complexities of diagnosis and treatment with confidence. Grant me discernment in providing the best care for my patients.

Prayer Request

_____

_____

_____

_____

DAY 22

Dear God,

When I feel overwhelmed, remind me of the importance of self-care. Guide me towards activities that bring me joy and peace, whether it be spending time in nature, pursuing hobbies, or connecting with loved ones.

Prayer Request

_____

_____

_____

_____

DAY 23

Heavenly Father,

I surrender my fears and anxieties about the future to you. Help me live in the present moment, focusing on the lives I can touch today. Fill me with hope for a brighter tomorrow.

Prayer Request

DAY 24

Dear God,

As I begin this day, I release any negative thoughts that weigh me down. Replace them with thoughts of gratitude and positivity. Help me cultivate a mindset of resilience and optimism.

Prayer Request

_____

_____

_____

_____

DAY 25

Dear Father,

I pray for emotional healing from the wounds that depression has caused. Restore my joy and enthusiasm for life. Renew my spirit and remind me of the incredible privilege it is to serve as a doctor.

Prayer Request

DAY 26

Heavenly Father,

Bless my interactions with patients today. Grant me the ability to listen deeply and empathize with their struggles. Let me be a source of comfort and support, showing them that they are not alone.

Prayer Request

_____

_____

_____

_____

DAY 27

Dear Lord,

When I feel discouraged or defeated, remind me of the lives I have touched and the difference I have made. Allow me to see the ripple effect of my actions and the lasting impact I have on individuals and communities.

Prayer Request

DAY 28

Dear God,

I surrender my need for control and perfection. Help me embrace the uncertainties of my profession and trust in your divine guidance. Fill me with courage and resilience to face whatever comes my way.

Prayer Request

DAY 29

Dear Father,

I pray for open doors and new opportunities to bring healing and hope. Guide me to avenues where I can make a difference beyond the confines of my medical practice. Inspire me to be a catalyst for positive change.

Prayer Request

DAY 30

Dear God,

I pray for a renewed sense of purpose and meaning in my work. Remind me of the lives I have saved, the families I have comforted, and the impact I have made. Let me never lose sight of the noble calling of medicine.

Prayer Request

_____

_____

_____

_____